FERTILITY DIET FOR OLDER WOMEN

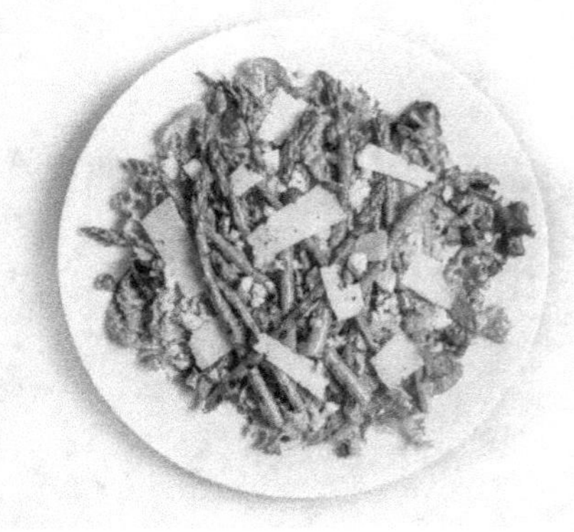

DR. JESSICA SMITH

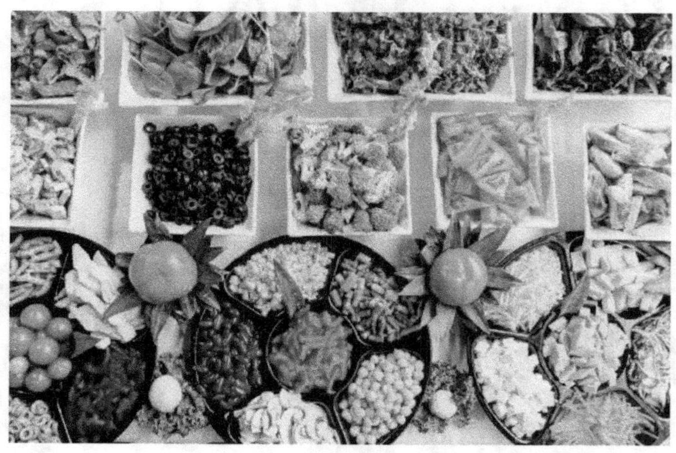

TABLE OF CONTENTS

CHAPTER ONE

How to Use this Cookbook

Prioritize Nutrient-Rich Foods: Focus on a diet rich in fruits, vegetables, whole grains, lean proteins, and healthy fats. These foods provide essential vitamins, minerals, and antioxidants crucial for reproductive health.

Include Folate-Rich Foods: Incorporate foods high in folate such as leafy greens, citrus fruits, legumes, and fortified grains. Folate supports healthy ovulation and reduces the risk of neural tube defects in newborns.

Opt for Lean Protein Sources: Choose lean protein sources such as poultry, fish, tofu, beans, and lentils. Protein is essential for hormone production and egg quality.

Consume Healthy Fats: Include sources of healthy fats like avocados, nuts, seeds, and olive oil in your diet. Healthy fats support hormone balance and reproductive function.

Limit Processed Foods and Added Sugars: Minimize intake of processed foods, sugary snacks, and beverages. These can lead to inflammation and hormonal imbalances, negatively impacting fertility.

Stay Hydrated: Drink plenty of water throughout the day to stay hydrated. Proper hydration supports overall health and helps maintain cervical mucus consistency, which is important for conception.

Monitor Caffeine Intake: Limit caffeine consumption to moderate levels, as excessive caffeine intake may interfere with fertility. Stick to one to two cups of coffee per day, or opt for caffeine-free alternatives.

Include Iron-Rich Foods: Incorporate iron-rich foods such as lean meats, leafy greens, beans, and fortified cereals to prevent iron deficiency anemia, which can affect fertility and pregnancy outcomes.

Maintain a Healthy Weight: Aim for a healthy weight through balanced nutrition and regular physical activity. Excess weight can disrupt hormone levels and menstrual cycles, while being underweight may affect ovulation.

Consider Supplements: Consult with a healthcare provider about taking prenatal vitamins or specific supplements tailored to support fertility, such as omega-3 fatty acids, vitamin D, and Coenzyme Q10.

Understanding the unique needs of older women in relation to fertility and diet is crucial for optimizing reproductive health and increasing the likelihood of conception.

As women age, various factors such as declining egg quality, decreased ovarian reserve, and hormonal changes can affect fertility.

However, adopting a fertility-focused diet tailored to the needs of older women can help mitigate these challenges and support a healthy reproductive system.

A fertility diet for older women emphasizes nutrient-dense foods that provide essential vitamins, minerals, and antioxidants necessary for optimal fertility.

This includes a variety of fruits, vegetables, whole grains, lean proteins, and healthy fats. Key nutrients such as folate, iron, omega-3 fatty acids, and vitamin D play important roles in supporting egg quality, hormone balance, and overall reproductive function.

Additionally, older women may benefit from limiting their intake of processed foods, added sugars, and unhealthy fats, as these can contribute to inflammation and hormonal imbalances that may negatively impact fertility.

Maintaining a healthy weight through balanced nutrition and regular physical activity is also important, as excess weight or being underweight can affect hormone levels and menstrual cycles.

By focusing on nutrient-rich foods, staying hydrated, managing caffeine intake, and considering supplements when necessary, older women can optimize their fertility and increase their chances of conceiving a healthy pregnancy.

It's essential for older women to work closely with healthcare providers or fertility specialists to develop a personalized fertility diet plan that addresses their specific needs and goals.

Principles of Fertility Diet for Older Women

The principles of a fertility diet for older women are centered around supporting reproductive health, addressing age-related factors that may impact fertility, and optimizing the chances of conception.

- **Here are the key principles:**

Nutrient-Rich Foods: Emphasize a diet rich in nutrient-dense foods such as fruits, vegetables, whole grains, lean proteins, and healthy fats. These foods provide essential vitamins, minerals, antioxidants, and phytonutrients necessary for optimal fertility.

Folate and B Vitamins: Incorporate foods high in folate and B vitamins, such as leafy greens, legumes, fortified grains, and nuts. Folate is crucial for healthy egg development, DNA synthesis, and reducing the risk of neural tube defects in the developing fetus.

Healthy Fats: Include sources of healthy fats like avocados, nuts, seeds, and fatty fish. Omega-3 fatty acids support hormone balance, reduce inflammation, and promote optimal egg quality.

Protein: Choose lean protein sources such as poultry, fish, tofu, beans, and lentils. Protein is essential for hormone production, egg development, and overall reproductive function.

Limit Processed Foods and Added Sugars: Minimize intake of processed foods, sugary snacks, and beverages, as they can lead to inflammation, insulin resistance, and hormonal imbalances that may hinder fertility.

Hydration: Stay hydrated by drinking plenty of water throughout the day. Proper hydration supports cervical mucus production, which is essential for sperm motility and conception.

Maintain a Healthy Weight: Aim for a healthy weight through balanced nutrition and regular exercise. Excess weight or being underweight can impact hormone levels, menstrual cycles, and fertility.

Supplements: Consider taking prenatal vitamins or specific supplements such as omega-3 fatty acids, vitamin D, and Coenzyme Q10 under the guidance of a healthcare provider to support fertility.

By adhering to these principles of a fertility diet, older women can create an environment conducive to conception, optimize reproductive health, and increase the likelihood of achieving a healthy pregnancy.

It's important for older women to work closely with healthcare providers or fertility specialists to develop a personalized dietary plan tailored to their specific needs and goals.

Benefits of Fertility Diet for Older Women

The benefits of adopting a fertility diet for older women extend beyond just enhancing the chances of conception; it encompasses promoting overall reproductive health, addressing age-related fertility challenges, and supporting the development of a healthy pregnancy.

Here are some key benefits:

Optimized Egg Quality: A fertility diet rich in antioxidants, vitamins, and minerals can help improve egg quality, which tends to decline with age.

Nutrient-dense foods such as fruits, vegetables, and lean proteins provide essential nutrients that support egg development and reduce oxidative stress, potentially improving the chances of successful fertilization.

Balanced Hormones: Hormonal balance is critical for fertility, and certain nutrients play key roles in hormone production and regulation. The inclusion of healthy fats, such as omega-3 fatty acids found in fatty fish and nuts, can help support hormone synthesis and balance, which is particularly beneficial for older women experiencing hormonal fluctuations.

Reduced Inflammation: Chronic inflammation has been linked to various fertility issues, including ovulatory disorders and implantation failure. By focusing on anti-inflammatory foods like fruits, vegetables, and whole grains, a fertility diet can help reduce inflammation levels in the body, creating a more conducive environment for conception and pregnancy.

Improved Ovarian Function: Age-related decline in ovarian function is a common concern for older women trying to conceive. A diet rich in nutrients like folate, vitamin D, and iron can support ovarian health and function, potentially enhancing ovarian reserve and responsiveness to fertility treatments.

Enhanced Reproductive Health: Overall, adopting a fertility diet can contribute to enhanced reproductive health by providing the body with the necessary nutrients and support it needs for optimal function.

This not only improves the chances of conception but also lays the foundation for a healthy pregnancy and the birth of a healthy baby.

By nourishing the body with nutrient-dense foods and adopting healthy lifestyle habits, older women can increase their chances of achieving their dream of conception and parenthood.

Tips for Fertility Diet for Older Women

When considering a fertility diet tailored to older women, it's important to focus on nutrient-dense foods and lifestyle practices that support reproductive health and optimize the chances of conception.

Here are some tips for creating a fertility-friendly diet for older women:

Prioritize Whole Foods: Base your diet on whole, minimally processed foods such as fruits, vegetables, whole grains, lean proteins, and healthy fats.

These foods provide essential nutrients necessary for reproductive health and overall well-being.

Include Folate-Rich Foods: Incorporate foods high in folate such as leafy greens, legumes, fortified grains, and citrus fruits. Folate plays a crucial role in DNA synthesis, egg quality, and reducing the risk of neural tube defects in newborns.

Focus on Healthy Fats: Choose sources of healthy fats such as avocados, nuts, seeds, and fatty fish. Omega-3 fatty acids support hormone balance, reduce inflammation, and promote optimal egg quality.

Opt for Lean Proteins: Include lean protein sources like poultry, fish, tofu, beans, and lentils in your meals. Protein is essential for hormone production, egg development, and overall reproductive function.

Limit Processed Foods and Added Sugars: Minimize intake of processed foods, sugary snacks, and beverages, as they can lead to inflammation, insulin resistance, and hormonal imbalances that may hinder fertility.

Stay Hydrated: Drink plenty of water throughout the day to stay hydrated.

Proper hydration supports cervical mucus production, which is essential for sperm motility and conception.

Moderate Caffeine and Alcohol: Limit caffeine and alcohol intake, as excessive consumption may interfere with fertility. Stick to moderate amounts and consider switching to decaffeinated or herbal options.

Manage Stress: Practice stress-reducing techniques such as yoga, meditation, deep breathing exercises, or engaging in hobbies and activities you enjoy. Chronic stress can negatively impact hormone levels and fertility.

Maintain a Healthy Weight: Aim for a healthy weight through balanced nutrition and regular exercise. Excess weight or being underweight can affect hormone levels, menstrual cycles, and fertility.

Consult with a Healthcare Provider: Seek guidance from a healthcare provider or fertility specialist who can offer personalized advice and recommendations based on your individual health needs and goals.

By incorporating these tips into your lifestyle and dietary habits, you can create a fertility-friendly environment that supports optimal reproductive health and increases the likelihood of conception, even as you age.

Remember that consistency and patience are key, and it's essential to work closely with healthcare professionals to address any specific concerns or challenges you may encounter along the way.

Guidelines for Fertility Diet for Older Women

Guidelines for a fertility diet tailored to older women involve focusing on nutrient-dense foods, maintaining a healthy lifestyle, and addressing age-related factors that may impact reproductive health.

Here are some essential guidelines to consider:

Nutrient-Rich Foods: Base your diet on whole, minimally processed foods such as fruits, vegetables, whole grains, lean proteins, and healthy fats. These foods provide essential vitamins, minerals, antioxidants, and phytonutrients necessary for optimal fertility.

Folate and B Vitamins: Incorporate folate-rich foods such as leafy greens, legumes, fortified grains, and citrus fruits.

Folate supports healthy egg development, DNA synthesis, and reduces the risk of neural tube defects in newborns.

Healthy Fats: Include sources of healthy fats like avocados, nuts, seeds, and fatty fish. Omega-3 fatty acids support hormone balance, reduce inflammation, and promote optimal egg quality.

Lean Proteins: Choose lean protein sources such as poultry, fish, tofu, beans, and lentils. Protein is essential for hormone production, egg development, and overall reproductive function.

Limit Processed Foods and Added Sugars: Minimize intake of processed foods, sugary snacks, and beverages, as they can lead to inflammation, insulin resistance, and hormonal imbalances that may hinder fertility.

Hydration: Drink plenty of water throughout the day to stay hydrated. Proper hydration supports cervical mucus production, which is essential for sperm motility and conception.

Moderate Caffeine and Alcohol: Limit caffeine and alcohol intake, as excessive consumption may interfere with fertility. Stick to moderate amounts and consider switching to decaffeinated or herbal options.

Maintain a Healthy Weight: Aim for a healthy weight through balanced nutrition and regular exercise. Excess weight or being underweight can impact hormone levels, menstrual cycles, and fertility.

Manage Stress: Practice stress-reducing techniques such as yoga, meditation, deep breathing exercises, or engaging in hobbies and activities you enjoy. Chronic stress can negatively impact hormone levels and fertility.

Consult with Healthcare Providers: Seek guidance from healthcare providers or fertility specialists who can offer personalized advice and recommendations based on individual health needs and goals.

CHAPTER TWO

Fertility Diet Breakfast Recipes for Older Women

1. Berry Spinach Smoothie

Ingredients:

- 1 cup spinach
- 1/2 cup mixed berries (strawberries, blueberries, raspberries)
- 1/2 banana
- 1/2 cup Greek yogurt or almond milk
- 1 tablespoon chia seeds
- Optional: honey or maple syrup for sweetness

Instructions:

- Place all ingredients in a blender.
- Blend until smooth.
- Pour into a glass and enjoy!

Health Benefits:

- Spinach provides folate, iron, and antioxidants.
- Berries are rich in antioxidants and vitamin C.

➢ Chia seeds offer omega-3 fatty acids and fiber for hormone balance and satiety.

Preparation Time: 5 minutes

2. Avocado Toast with Poached Egg

Ingredients:

➢ 1 slice whole grain bread
➢ 1/2 ripe avocado
➢ 1 egg
➢ Salt and pepper to taste
➢ Optional: red pepper flakes or sliced tomatoes for topping

Instructions:

➢ Toast the bread to your desired level of crispiness.
➢ Mash the avocado and spread it evenly onto the toast.
➢ Poach the egg in simmering water until cooked to your liking.
➢ Place the poached egg on top of the avocado toast.
➢ Season with salt, pepper, and any additional toppings as desired.

Health Benefits:

> ➤ Avocado provides healthy fats and vitamin E.
> ➤ Eggs offer high-quality protein and essential nutrients like choline.
> ➤ Whole grain bread provides fiber for digestive health and sustained energy.

Preparation Time: 10 minutes

3. Greek Yogurt Parfait

Ingredients:

> ➤ 1/2 cup Greek yogurt
> ➤ 1/4 cup granola
> ➤ 1/2 cup mixed berries (strawberries, blueberries, raspberries)
> ➤ 1 tablespoon honey or maple syrup
> ➤ Optional: sliced almonds or walnuts for topping

Instructions:

> ➤ In a serving glass or bowl, layer Greek yogurt, granola, and mixed berries.
> ➤ Drizzle honey or maple syrup over the top.
> ➤ Sprinkle with sliced almonds or walnuts if desired.

➢ Repeat the layers if making multiple servings.

➢ Serve immediately and enjoy!

Health Benefits:

➢ Greek yogurt provides protein and probiotics for gut health.

➢ Granola offers fiber, healthy fats, and complex carbohydrates.

➢ Berries are rich in antioxidants and vitamin C, supporting fertility and overall health.

Preparation Time: 5 minutes

4. Quinoa Breakfast Bowl

Ingredients:

➢ 1/2 cup cooked quinoa

➢ 1/4 cup almond milk or Greek yogurt

➢ 1/2 banana, sliced

➢ 1 tablespoon almond butter or peanut butter

➢ 1 tablespoon chia seeds or ground flaxseeds

➢ Optional: honey or maple syrup for sweetness

Instructions:

> In a bowl, combine cooked quinoa with almond milk or Greek yogurt.
> Top with sliced banana, almond butter or peanut butter, and chia seeds or ground flaxseeds.
> Drizzle with honey or maple syrup if desired.
> Mix well and serve immediately.

Health Benefits:

> Quinoa provides protein, fiber, and essential nutrients like iron and magnesium.
> Almond butter or peanut butter offers healthy fats and protein.
> Chia seeds or ground flaxseeds provide omega-3 fatty acids and additional fiber for hormone balance and satiety.

Preparation Time: 10 minutes (if quinoa is pre-cooked)

5. Veggie Omelette

Ingredients:

> 2 eggs
> 1/4 cup diced bell peppers

- ➢ 1/4 cup diced tomatoes
- ➢ 1/4 cup chopped spinach
- ➢ Salt and pepper to taste
- ➢ Optional: shredded cheese or avocado for topping

Instructions:

- ➢ In a bowl, whisk the eggs until well beaten.
- ➢ Heat a non-stick skillet over medium heat and lightly coat with cooking spray or olive oil.
- ➢ Pour the beaten eggs into the skillet.
- ➢ Add diced bell peppers, tomatoes, and chopped spinach on one half of the omelette.
- ➢ Season with salt and pepper.
- ➢ Once the eggs start to set, fold the other half of the omelette over the filling.
- ➢ Cook for another 1-2 minutes until the omelette is fully cooked.
- ➢ Slide the omelette onto a plate and serve with shredded cheese or sliced avocado if desired.

Health Benefits:

- ➢ Eggs provide high-quality protein and essential nutrients like choline.

- ➤ Bell peppers, tomatoes, and spinach offer vitamins, minerals, and antioxidants.
- ➤ Avocado provides healthy fats and vitamin E.

Preparation Time: 10 minutes

6. Chia Seed Pudding

Ingredients:

- ➤ 1/4 cup chia seeds
- ➤ 1 cup almond milk or any plant-based milk
- ➤ 1 tablespoon maple syrup or sweetener of choice
- ➤ 1/2 teaspoon vanilla extract
- ➤ Toppings: sliced fruits, nuts, seeds, coconut flakes

Instructions:

- ➤ In a mason jar or airtight container, combine chia seeds, almond milk, maple syrup, and vanilla extract.
- ➤ Stir well to combine.
- ➤ Cover and refrigerate for at least 2 hours, or overnight, until the mixture thickens and forms a pudding-like consistency.
- ➤ Once the chia pudding is ready, give it a good stir.

- ➢ Serve chilled with toppings of choice, such as sliced fruits, nuts, seeds, and coconut flakes.

Health Benefits:

- ➢ Chia seeds are rich in omega-3 fatty acids, protein, and fiber, promoting heart health, satiety, and digestive health.
- ➢ Almond milk is low in calories and contains healthy fats and vitamin E.

Preparation Time: 5 minutes (plus chilling time)

7. Veggie Breakfast Burrito

Ingredients:

- ➢ 1 whole grain tortilla or wrap
- ➢ 1/2 cup tofu scramble (see recipe #3)
- ➢ 1/4 cup black beans, rinsed and drained
- ➢ 1/4 cup diced avocado
- ➢ Salsa or hot sauce (optional)
- ➢ Fresh cilantro for garnish
- ➢ Salt and pepper to taste

Instructions:

> Heat the tortilla or wrap in a skillet or microwave until warm and pliable.
> Spread tofu scramble onto the tortilla, leaving space around the edges.
> Top with black beans, diced avocado, salsa or hot sauce (if using), and fresh cilantro.
> Season with salt and pepper to taste.
> Fold in the sides of the tortilla and roll it up tightly to form a burrito.
> Serve immediately.

Health Benefits:

> Tofu provides plant-based protein and essential amino acids, supporting muscle repair and satiety.
> Black beans are a good source of protein, fiber, and antioxidants, promoting heart health and blood sugar control.
> Avocado adds healthy fats, fiber, and vitamins, supporting heart health and satiety.

Preparation Time: 15 minutes (if tofu scramble is pre-made)

8. Green Smoothie

Ingredients:

- 1 cup spinach or kale leaves
- 1/2 frozen banana
- 1/2 cup frozen mixed berries
- 1/4 avocado
- 1 tablespoon chia seeds
- 1 cup almond milk or any plant-based milk

Instructions:

- Place all ingredients in a blender.
- Blend until smooth and creamy.
- If the smoothie is too thick, add more almond milk as needed.
- Pour into a glass and enjoy!

Health Benefits:

- Spinach or kale provides folate, iron, and antioxidants.
- Berries offer antioxidants and vitamin C, supporting immune function and fertility.
- Avocado provides healthy fats and vitamin E.

➤ Chia seeds offer omega-3 fatty acids and fiber for satiety and digestive health.

Preparation Time: 5 minutes

9. Overnight Oats

Ingredients:

➤ 1/2 cup rolled oats

➤ 1/2 cup almond milk or any plant-based milk

➤ 1/2 cup Greek yogurt

➤ 1 tablespoon chia seeds

➤ 1/2 teaspoon vanilla extract

➤ Toppings: sliced fruits, nuts, seeds, honey or maple syrup

Instructions:

➤ In a mason jar or airtight container, combine rolled oats, almond milk, Greek yogurt, chia seeds, and vanilla extract.

➤ Stir well to combine.

➤ Cover and refrigerate overnight, or for at least 4 hours.

➤ Once the oats are ready, give them a good stir.

> Serve cold with toppings of choice, such as sliced fruits, nuts, seeds, and honey or maple syrup.

Health Benefits:

> Rolled oats provide fiber, complex carbohydrates, and essential nutrients like iron and magnesium, supporting heart health and digestive health.
> Greek yogurt offers protein, probiotics, and calcium, promoting gut health and bone health.
> Chia seeds provide omega-3 fatty acids, fiber, and antioxidants, supporting heart health, satiety, and digestive health.

Preparation Time: 5 minutes (plus chilling time)

10. Whole Grain Pancakes

Ingredients:

> 1/2 cup whole wheat flour or oat flour
> 1/2 teaspoon baking powder
> Pinch of salt
> 1/2 cup almond milk or any plant-based milk
> 1 egg
> 1 tablespoon maple syrup or sweetener of choice

- ➢ 1/2 teaspoon vanilla extract
- ➢ Cooking spray or olive oil for greasing the skillet
- ➢ Toppings: sliced fruits, nuts, seeds, honey or maple syrup

Instructions:

- ➢ In a mixing bowl, combine whole wheat flour, baking powder, and salt.
- ➢ In a separate bowl, whisk together almond milk, egg, maple syrup, and vanilla extract.
- ➢ Pour the wet ingredients into the dry ingredients and stir until just combined. Be careful not to overmix.
- ➢ Heat a non-stick skillet over medium heat and lightly coat with cooking spray or olive oil.
- ➢ Pour 1/4 cup of batter onto the skillet for each pancake.
- ➢ Cook until bubbles form on the surface of the pancake, then flip and cook until golden brown on the other side.
- ➢ Repeat with the remaining batter.
- ➢ Serve pancakes warm with toppings of choice, such as sliced fruits, nuts, seeds, and honey or maple syrup.

Health Benefits:

> Whole wheat flour or oat flour provides fiber, vitamins, and minerals, supporting heart health and digestive health.
> Almond milk offers fewer calories than cow's milk and contains healthy fats and vitamin E.
> Eggs provide high-quality protein and essential nutrients like choline.

Preparation Time: 15 minutes

Fertility Diet Lunch Recipes for Older Women

1. Quinoa Salad with Roasted Vegetables

Ingredients:

> 1 cup quinoa
> Assorted vegetables (such as bell peppers, zucchini, cherry tomatoes)
> Olive oil
> Salt and pepper
> Fresh herbs (such as parsley or basil)
> Lemon juice

Instructions:

- ➢ Cook quinoa according to package instructions.
- ➢ Preheat oven to 400°F (200°C). Chop vegetables and toss with olive oil, salt, and pepper. Roast in the oven for 20-25 minutes until tender and slightly caramelized.
- ➢ In a large bowl, combine cooked quinoa and roasted vegetables. Drizzle with lemon juice, add fresh herbs, and toss to combine.
- ➢ Serve warm or at room temperature.

Health Benefits:

- ➢ Quinoa is a complete protein, providing essential amino acids necessary for hormone production and reproductive health.
- ➢ Vegetables are rich in vitamins, minerals, and antioxidants, supporting overall health and fertility.
- ➢ Olive oil offers healthy fats, which are important for hormone balance and reproductive function.

Preparation Time: 30 minutes

2. Lentil Soup

Ingredients:

- 1 cup dried lentils
- 4 cups vegetable broth
- Assorted vegetables (such as carrots, celery, onions)
- Garlic cloves, minced
- Bay leaves
- Herbs and spices (such as thyme, rosemary, paprika)
- Salt and pepper to taste

Instructions:

- Rinse lentils under cold water and drain.
- In a large pot, sauté minced garlic, chopped vegetables, and herbs in olive oil until softened.
- Add lentils, vegetable broth, bay leaves, and seasonings to the pot. Bring to a boil, then reduce heat and simmer for 25-30 minutes until lentils are tender.
- Remove bay leaves and adjust seasoning if necessary.
- Serve hot, garnished with fresh herbs if desired.

Health Benefits:

> Lentils are a good source of plant-based protein, fiber, and folate, supporting hormone balance and reproductive health.
> Vegetables provide essential nutrients and antioxidants, promoting overall health and fertility.
> Garlic and herbs offer anti-inflammatory and immune-boosting properties.

Preparation Time: 40 minutes

3. Salmon and Quinoa Bowl

Ingredients:

> 1 fillet of salmon
> 1/2 cup quinoa
> Assorted vegetables (such as spinach, cherry tomatoes, cucumbers)
> Lemon wedges
> Olive oil
> Salt and pepper

Instructions:

> Cook quinoa according to package instructions.

- ➢ Preheat oven to 400°F (200°C). Season salmon fillet with olive oil, salt, and pepper. Bake in the oven for 12-15 minutes until cooked through.
- ➢ Assemble bowls with cooked quinoa, assorted vegetables, and baked salmon.
- ➢ Serve with lemon wedges and a drizzle of olive oil.

Health Benefits:

- ➢ Salmon is rich in omega-3 fatty acids, protein, and vitamin D, supporting hormone balance and reproductive function.
- ➢ Quinoa provides protein, fiber, and essential nutrients necessary for fertility.
- ➢ Vegetables offer vitamins, minerals, and antioxidants, promoting overall health and reproductive wellness.

Preparation Time: 30 minutes

4. Chickpea and Avocado Wrap

Ingredients:

- ➢ 1 whole grain tortilla or wrap
- ➢ 1/2 cup cooked chickpeas

- ➤ 1/4 avocado, mashed
- ➤ Assorted vegetables (such as lettuce, tomatoes, bell peppers)
- ➤ Hummus (optional)
- ➤ Lemon juice
- ➤ Salt and pepper

Instructions:

- ➤ In a small bowl, mash chickpeas with mashed avocado, lemon juice, salt, and pepper.
- ➤ Spread hummus (if using) on the tortilla or wrap.
- ➤ Layer mashed chickpea and avocado mixture onto the tortilla, along with assorted vegetables.
- ➤ Roll up the tortilla tightly to form a wrap.
- ➤ Serve immediately or wrap in foil for later.

Health Benefits:

- ➤ Chickpeas provide plant-based protein, fiber, and folate, supporting hormone balance and reproductive health.
- ➤ Avocado offers healthy fats, vitamins, and minerals, promoting fertility and overall wellness.

- ➢ Whole grain tortillas provide complex carbohydrates and fiber, sustaining energy levels and supporting reproductive function.

Preparation Time: 15 minutes

5. Tofu Stir-Fry

Ingredients:

- ➢ 1 block of firm tofu, cubed
- ➢ Assorted vegetables (such as broccoli, bell peppers, snap peas)
- ➢ Garlic cloves, minced
- ➢ Ginger, grated
- ➢ Soy sauce or tamari
- ➢ Sesame oil
- ➢ Rice vinegar
- ➢ Brown rice or quinoa

Instructions:

- ➢ Cook brown rice or quinoa according to package instructions.

- In a large skillet or wok, heat sesame oil over medium-high heat. Add minced garlic and grated ginger, and sauté until fragrant.
- Add cubed tofu to the skillet and cook until golden brown on all sides.
- Add assorted vegetables to the skillet and stir-fry until tender-crisp.
- Season with soy sauce or tamari and rice vinegar, adjusting to taste.
- Serve tofu stir-fry over cooked brown rice or quinoa.

Health Benefits:

- Tofu provides plant-based protein, calcium, and iron, supporting hormone balance and reproductive health.
- Assorted vegetables offer vitamins, minerals, and antioxidants, promoting overall health and fertility.
- Brown rice or quinoa provides complex carbohydrates and fiber, supporting energy levels and reproductive function.

Preparation Time: 30 minutes

6. Spinach and Mushroom Omelette

Ingredients:

- ➢ 2 eggs
- ➢ Handful of spinach leaves
- ➢ Sliced mushrooms
- ➢ Onion, diced
- ➢ Olive oil
- ➢ Salt and pepper
- ➢ Fresh herbs (such as parsley or chives)

Instructions:

- ➢ In a bowl, whisk eggs until well beaten. Season with salt and pepper.
- ➢ Heat olive oil in a skillet over medium heat. Add diced onion and sliced mushrooms, and sauté until softened.
- ➢ Add spinach leaves to the skillet and cook until wilted.
- ➢ Pour beaten eggs into the skillet, swirling to cover the vegetables evenly.
- ➢ Cook until the omelette is set and the edges start to lift from the skillet.

- ➢ Carefully fold the omelette in half and transfer to a plate.
- ➢ Garnish with fresh herbs and serve hot.

Health Benefits:

- ➢ Eggs provide high-quality protein, vitamins, and minerals, supporting hormone balance and reproductive health.
- ➢ Spinach is rich in iron, folate, and antioxidants, promoting fertility and overall wellness.
- ➢ Mushrooms offer nutrients like vitamin D and selenium, supporting immune function and reproductive health.

Preparation Time: 15 minutes

7. Mediterranean Chickpea Salad

Ingredients:

- ➢ 1 can (15 ounces) chickpeas, drained and rinsed
- ➢ Cherry tomatoes, halved
- ➢ Cucumber, diced
- ➢ Red onion, thinly sliced
- ➢ Kalamata olives, pitted and halved

- ➤ Fresh parsley, chopped
- ➤ Feta cheese, crumbled (optional)
- ➤ Olive oil
- ➤ Lemon juice
- ➤ Garlic, minced
- ➤ Dried oregano
- ➤ Salt and pepper

Instructions:

- ➤ In a large bowl, combine chickpeas, cherry tomatoes, cucumber, red onion, olives, and parsley.
- ➤ In a small bowl, whisk together olive oil, lemon juice, minced garlic, dried oregano, salt, and pepper to make the dressing.
- ➤ Pour the dressing over the salad and toss to coat evenly.
- ➤ Sprinkle crumbled feta cheese on top if desired.
- ➤ Serve chilled or at room temperature.

Health Benefits:

- ➤ Chickpeas provide plant-based protein, fiber, and folate, supporting hormone balance and reproductive health.

- ➤ Vegetables offer vitamins, minerals, and antioxidants, promoting overall health and fertility.
- ➤ Olive oil provides healthy fats, which are important for hormone production and reproductive function.

Preparation Time: 15 minutes

8. Sweet Potato and Black Bean Bowl

Ingredients:

- ➤ 1 medium sweet potato, cubed
- ➤ 1 can (15 ounces) black beans, drained and rinsed
- ➤ Red bell pepper, diced
- ➤ Red onion, diced
- ➤ Avocado, sliced
- ➤ Fresh cilantro, chopped
- ➤ Lime wedges
- ➤ Olive oil
- ➤ Chili powder
- ➤ Cumin
- ➤ Salt and pepper

Instructions:

- ➤ Preheat oven to 400°F (200°C). Toss cubed sweet potato with olive oil, chili powder, cumin, salt, and pepper. Roast in the oven for 20-25 minutes until tender and slightly caramelized.
- ➤ In a bowl, combine roasted sweet potato, black beans, diced red bell pepper, and diced red onion.
- ➤ Drizzle with olive oil and lime juice, and sprinkle with fresh cilantro.
- ➤ Serve with sliced avocado and lime wedges.

Health Benefits:

- ➤ Sweet potatoes are rich in beta-carotene, vitamin C, and fiber, supporting hormone balance and reproductive health.
- ➤ Black beans provide plant-based protein, fiber, and folate, promoting fertility and overall wellness.
- ➤ Avocado offers healthy fats, vitamins, and minerals, which are important for reproductive function and fetal development.

Preparation Time: 30 minutes

9. Greek Yogurt Parfait

Ingredients:

> Greek yogurt

> Mixed berries (such as strawberries, blueberries, raspberries)

> Granola

> Honey (optional)

Instructions:

> In a glass or bowl, layer Greek yogurt, mixed berries, and granola.

> Drizzle with honey if desired.

> Repeat the layers until the glass or bowl is filled.

> Serve immediately as a nutritious and satisfying lunch or snack option.

Health Benefits:

> Greek yogurt is rich in protein, calcium, and probiotics, supporting hormone balance and reproductive health.

> Mixed berries offer antioxidants, vitamins, and fiber, promoting fertility and overall wellness.

➤ Granola provides complex carbohydrates and fiber, sustaining energy levels and supporting reproductive function.

Preparation Time: 5 minutes

10. Veggie and Hummus Wrap

Ingredients:

➤ 1 whole grain tortilla or wrap

➤ Hummus

➤ Assorted vegetables (such as lettuce, shredded carrots, cucumber slices, bell peppers)

➤ Sprouts or microgreens

➤ Lemon juice

➤ Salt and pepper

Instructions:

➤ Spread a layer of hummus on the tortilla or wrap.

➤ Layer assorted vegetables and sprouts or microgreens on top of the hummus.

➤ Drizzle with lemon juice and season with salt and pepper to taste.

➤ Roll up the tortilla tightly to form a wrap.

> Serve immediately or wrap in foil for later.

Health Benefits:

> Hummus provides plant-based protein, fiber, and healthy fats, supporting hormone balance and reproductive health.
> Assorted vegetables offer vitamins, minerals, and antioxidants, promoting overall health and fertility.
> Whole grain tortillas provide complex carbohydrates and fiber, sustaining energy levels and supporting reproductive function.

Preparation Time: 10 minutes

Fertility Diet Dinner Recipes for Older Women

1. Baked Salmon with Asparagus and Quinoa

Ingredients:

> 1 salmon fillet
> Asparagus spears
> Olive oil
> Salt and pepper
> Lemon wedges
> Quinoa

- ➢ Fresh dill (optional)

Instructions:

- ➢ Preheat oven to 400°F (200°C). Place salmon fillet on a baking sheet lined with parchment paper.
- ➢ Drizzle salmon with olive oil and season with salt and pepper. Place asparagus spears around the salmon.
- ➢ Bake in the oven for 12-15 minutes until salmon is cooked through and asparagus is tender.
- ➢ Meanwhile, cook quinoa according to package instructions.
- ➢ Serve baked salmon and asparagus over cooked quinoa, garnished with fresh dill and lemon wedges.

Health Benefits:

- ➢ Salmon provides omega-3 fatty acids and protein, supporting hormone balance and reproductive health.
- ➢ Asparagus offers folate, fiber, and antioxidants, promoting fertility and overall wellness.
- ➢ Quinoa provides protein, fiber, and essential nutrients necessary for optimal fertility.

Preparation Time: 25 minutes

2. Lentil and Vegetable Stir-Fry

Ingredients:

> 1 cup dried lentils

> Assorted vegetables (such as broccoli, bell peppers, carrots)

> Garlic cloves, minced

> Ginger, grated

> Soy sauce or tamari

> Sesame oil

> Rice vinegar

> Brown rice

> Green onions, chopped (optional)

Instructions:

> Rinse lentils under cold water and drain. Cook lentils according to package instructions.

> In a large skillet or wok, heat sesame oil over medium-high heat. Add minced garlic and grated ginger, and sauté until fragrant.

> Add assorted vegetables to the skillet and stir-fry until tender-crisp.

- ➢ Add cooked lentils to the skillet and stir to combine. Season with soy sauce or tamari and rice vinegar, adjusting to taste.
- ➢ Serve lentil and vegetable stir-fry over cooked brown rice, garnished with chopped green onions if desired.

Health Benefits:

- ➢ Lentils provide plant-based protein, fiber, and folate, supporting hormone balance and reproductive health.
- ➢ Vegetables offer vitamins, minerals, and antioxidants, promoting overall health and fertility.
- ➢ Brown rice provides complex carbohydrates and fiber, supporting energy levels and reproductive function.

Preparation Time: 30 minutes

3. Grilled Chicken and Vegetable Skewers

Ingredients:

- ➢ Chicken breast, cut into cubes
- ➢ Assorted vegetables (such as cherry tomatoes, bell peppers, zucchini)

- Olive oil
- Garlic powder
- Italian seasoning
- Salt and pepper
- Lemon wedges

Instructions:

- Preheat grill to medium-high heat.
- Thread chicken cubes and assorted vegetables onto skewers.
- Drizzle skewers with olive oil and sprinkle with garlic powder, Italian seasoning, salt, and pepper.
- Grill skewers for 10-12 minutes, turning occasionally, until chicken is cooked through and vegetables are tender.
- Serve grilled chicken and vegetable skewers with lemon wedges for squeezing over the top.

Health Benefits:

- Chicken provides lean protein and essential amino acids, supporting hormone balance and reproductive health.

- ➤ Vegetables offer vitamins, minerals, and antioxidants, promoting overall health and fertility.
- ➤ Olive oil provides healthy fats, which are important for hormone production and reproductive function.

Preparation Time: 20 minutes

4. Veggie and Bean Burrito Bowl

Ingredients:

- ➤ Cooked brown rice
- ➤ Black beans, cooked and seasoned
- ➤ Assorted vegetables (such as lettuce, diced tomatoes, corn, avocado)
- ➤ Salsa
- ➤ Guacamole
- ➤ Cilantro, chopped
- ➤ Lime wedges

Instructions:

- ➤ Divide cooked brown rice among serving bowls.
- ➤ Top with seasoned black beans, assorted vegetables, salsa, and guacamole.

- ➢ Garnish with chopped cilantro and serve with lime wedges for squeezing over the top.
- ➢ Alternatively, assemble ingredients in a tortilla for a burrito.

Health Benefits:

- ➢ Brown rice provides complex carbohydrates and fiber, sustaining energy levels and supporting reproductive function.
- ➢ Black beans offer plant-based protein, fiber, and folate, promoting hormone balance and reproductive health.
- ➢ Assorted vegetables provide vitamins, minerals, and antioxidants, promoting overall health and fertility.

Preparation Time: 20 minutes

5. Turkey and Vegetable Stir-Fry

Ingredients:

- ➢ Ground turkey
- ➢ Assorted vegetables (such as broccoli, snap peas, bell peppers)
- ➢ Garlic cloves, minced

- ➤ Ginger, grated
- ➤ Soy sauce or tamari
- ➤ Sesame oil
- ➤ Rice vinegar
- ➤ Brown rice or quinoa

Instructions:

- ➤ Cook ground turkey in a skillet over medium heat until browned and cooked through.
- ➤ Add minced garlic and grated ginger to the skillet, and sauté until fragrant.
- ➤ Add assorted vegetables to the skillet and stir-fry until tender-crisp.
- ➤ In a small bowl, whisk together soy sauce or tamari, sesame oil, and rice vinegar. Pour over the turkey and vegetable mixture, and stir to combine.
- ➤ Serve turkey and vegetable stir-fry over cooked brown rice or quinoa.

Health Benefits:

- ➤ Turkey provides lean protein and essential amino acids, supporting hormone balance and reproductive health.

- ➢ Assorted vegetables offer vitamins, minerals, and antioxidants, promoting overall health and fertility.

- ➢ Brown rice or quinoa provides complex carbohydrates and fiber, sustaining energy levels and supporting reproductive function.

Preparation Time: 25 minutes

6. Eggplant and Chickpea Curry

Ingredients:

- ➢ Eggplant, cubed
- ➢ Cooked chickpeas
- ➢ Onion, diced
- ➢ Garlic cloves, minced
- ➢ Ginger, grated
- ➢ Curry powder
- ➢ Coconut milk
- ➢ Olive oil
- ➢ Fresh cilantro, chopped
- ➢ Cooked brown rice or quinoa

Instructions:

➢ In a large skillet, heat olive oil over medium heat. Add diced onion, minced garlic, and grated ginger, and sauté until softened.

➢ Add cubed eggplant to the skillet and cook until browned and softened.

➢ Stir in cooked chickpeas and curry powder, and cook for a few minutes until fragrant.

➢ Pour in coconut milk and simmer for 10-15 minutes until the curry has thickened and the flavors have melded.

➢ Serve eggplant and chickpea curry over cooked brown rice or quinoa, garnished with chopped fresh cilantro.

Health Benefits:

➢ Eggplant provides fiber, vitamins, and antioxidants, supporting overall health and fertility.

➢ Chickpeas offer plant-based protein, fiber, and folate, promoting hormone balance and reproductive health.

- ➢ Coconut milk provides healthy fats and adds creaminess to the curry, enhancing flavor and texture.

Preparation Time: 40 minutes

7. Shrimp and Vegetable Stir-Fry

Ingredients:

- ➢ Shrimp, peeled and deveined
- ➢ Assorted vegetables (such as broccoli, bell peppers, snap peas)
- ➢ Garlic cloves, minced
- ➢ Ginger, grated
- ➢ Soy sauce or tamari
- ➢ Sesame oil
- ➢ Rice vinegar
- ➢ Brown rice or quinoa

Instructions:

- ➢ Cook brown rice or quinoa according to package instructions.

- In a large skillet or wok, heat sesame oil over medium-high heat. Add minced garlic and grated ginger, and sauté until fragrant.
- Add shrimp to the skillet and cook until pink and cooked through. Remove from skillet and set aside.
- Add assorted vegetables to the skillet and stir-fry until tender-crisp.
- Return cooked shrimp to the skillet. In a small bowl, whisk together soy sauce or tamari, sesame oil, and rice vinegar. Pour over the shrimp and vegetable mixture, and stir to combine.
- Serve shrimp and vegetable stir-fry over cooked brown rice or quinoa.

Health Benefits:

- Shrimp provides lean protein and essential nutrients such as selenium and iodine, supporting hormone balance and reproductive health.
- Assorted vegetables offer vitamins, minerals, and antioxidants, promoting overall health and fertility.
- Brown rice or quinoa provides complex carbohydrates and fiber, sustaining energy levels and supporting reproductive function.

Preparation Time: 25 minutes

8. Spinach and Feta Stuffed Chicken Breast

Ingredients:

- Chicken breasts
- Fresh spinach leaves
- Feta cheese, crumbled
- Garlic cloves, minced
- Olive oil
- Salt and pepper
- Lemon wedges

Instructions:

- Preheat oven to 375°F (190°C). Using a sharp knife, make a horizontal slit in each chicken breast to create a pocket.
- In a small bowl, mix together crumbled feta cheese, minced garlic, and olive oil. Stuff the spinach leaves and feta mixture into the pockets of the chicken breasts.
- Season the outside of the chicken breasts with salt and pepper.

- ➢ Place stuffed chicken breasts on a baking sheet lined with parchment paper. Bake in the oven for 25-30 minutes until chicken is cooked through and juices run clear.
- ➢ Serve stuffed chicken breasts with lemon wedges for squeezing over the top.

Health Benefits:

- ➢ Chicken breasts provide lean protein and essential amino acids, supporting hormone balance and reproductive health.
- ➢ Spinach offers iron, folate, and antioxidants, promoting fertility and overall wellness.
- ➢ Feta cheese provides calcium and protein, contributing to bone health and reproductive function.

Preparation Time: 35 minutes

9. Tofu and Vegetable Stir-Fry with Brown Rice

Ingredients:

- ➢ Firm tofu, cubed

- ➢ Assorted vegetables (such as broccoli, bell peppers, carrots)
- ➢ Garlic cloves, minced
- ➢ Ginger, grated
- ➢ Soy sauce or tamari
- ➢ Sesame oil
- ➢ Rice vinegar
- ➢ Brown rice

Instructions:

- ➢ Cook brown rice according to package instructions.
- ➢ In a large skillet or wok, heat sesame oil over medium-high heat. Add minced garlic and grated ginger, and sauté until fragrant.
- ➢ Add cubed tofu to the skillet and cook until golden brown on all sides. Remove tofu from skillet and set aside.
- ➢ Add assorted vegetables to the skillet and stir-fry until tender-crisp.
- ➢ Return cooked tofu to the skillet. In a small bowl, whisk together soy sauce or tamari, sesame oil, and rice vinegar. Pour over the tofu and vegetable mixture, and stir to combine.

> Serve tofu and vegetable stir-fry over cooked brown rice.

Health Benefits:

> Tofu provides plant-based protein, calcium, and iron, supporting hormone balance and reproductive health.
> Assorted vegetables offer vitamins, minerals, and antioxidants, promoting overall health and fertility.
> Brown rice provides complex carbohydrates and fiber, sustaining energy levels and supporting reproductive function.

Preparation Time: 30 minutes

10. Mediterranean Stuffed Bell Peppers

Ingredients:

> Bell peppers
> Cooked quinoa or brown rice
> Chickpeas, cooked and seasoned
> Cherry tomatoes, halved
> Red onion, diced
> Kalamata olives, pitted and halved

- ➢ Feta cheese, crumbled

- ➢ Olive oil

- ➢ Lemon juice

- ➢ Fresh parsley, chopped

- ➢ Salt and pepper

Instructions:

- ➢ Preheat oven to 375°F (190°C). Cut the tops off the bell peppers and remove seeds and membranes.

- ➢ In a large bowl, combine cooked quinoa or brown rice, seasoned chickpeas, halved cherry tomatoes, diced red onion, halved Kalamata olives, crumbled feta cheese, olive oil, lemon juice, chopped parsley, salt, and pepper.

- ➢ Stuff the mixture into the bell peppers, pressing down gently to pack.

- ➢ Place stuffed bell peppers in a baking dish and cover with foil. Bake in the oven for 25-30 minutes until peppers are tender.

- ➢ Serve Mediterranean stuffed bell peppers hot, garnished with additional chopped parsley if desired.

Health Benefits:

> ➢ Bell peppers provide vitamin C and antioxidants, supporting fertility and overall health.
> ➢ Quinoa or brown rice offers complex carbohydrates and fiber, sustaining energy levels and supporting reproductive function.
> ➢ Chickpeas provide plant-based protein, fiber, and folate, promoting hormone balance and reproductive health.

Preparation Time: 40 minutes

Fertility Diet Snacks Recipes for Older Women

1. Berry Smoothie Bowl

Ingredients:

> ➢ 1 cup mixed berries (such as strawberries, blueberries, raspberries)
> ➢ 1 ripe banana
> ➢ 1/2 cup Greek yogurt
> ➢ 1/4 cup almond milk or coconut water
> ➢ 1 tablespoon chia seeds

- ➢ Honey or maple syrup (optional)
- ➢ Toppings: sliced almonds, shredded coconut, granola

Instructions:

- ➢ In a blender, combine mixed berries, banana, Greek yogurt, almond milk or coconut water, and chia seeds.
- ➢ Blend until smooth and creamy, adding honey or maple syrup if desired for sweetness.
- ➢ Pour the smoothie into a bowl and top with sliced almonds, shredded coconut, and granola.
- ➢ Enjoy with a spoon as a delicious and nutritious snack.

Health Benefits:

- ➢ Berries are rich in antioxidants, vitamins, and fiber, supporting fertility and overall wellness.
- ➢ Greek yogurt provides protein, calcium, and probiotics, promoting hormone balance and reproductive health.
- ➢ Chia seeds offer omega-3 fatty acids, fiber, and essential nutrients, supporting reproductive function and hormonal balance.

Preparation Time: 10 minutes

2. Avocado Toast

Ingredients:

- ➢ Whole grain bread or toast
- ➢ Ripe avocado
- ➢ Lemon juice
- ➢ Salt and pepper
- ➢ Optional toppings: sliced tomatoes, radishes, microgreens, hemp seeds

Instructions:

- ➢ Toast whole grain bread until golden brown and crispy.
- ➢ Mash ripe avocado with lemon juice, salt, and pepper.
- ➢ Spread avocado mixture onto the toasted bread.
- ➢ Top with sliced tomatoes, radishes, microgreens, or hemp seeds if desired.
- ➢ Serve immediately as a nutritious and satisfying snack option.

Health Benefits:

> ➤ Avocado offers healthy fats, vitamins, and minerals, supporting hormone balance and reproductive function.

> ➤ Whole grain bread provides complex carbohydrates and fiber, sustaining energy levels and supporting reproductive health.

> ➤ Optional toppings add vitamins, minerals, and antioxidants, promoting overall wellness and fertility.

Preparation Time: 5 minutes

3. Greek Yogurt with Honey and Almonds

Ingredients:

> ➤ Greek yogurt

> ➤ Raw almonds

> ➤ Honey

Instructions:

> ➤ Spoon Greek yogurt into a bowl.

> ➤ Drizzle with honey and sprinkle with raw almonds.

> ➤ Enjoy immediately as a quick and nutritious snack.

Health Benefits:

- ➢ Greek yogurt provides protein, calcium, and probiotics, supporting hormone balance and reproductive health.
- ➢ Raw almonds offer healthy fats, protein, and essential nutrients, promoting fertility and overall wellness.
- ➢ Honey adds natural sweetness and antioxidants, enhancing the flavor and nutritional value of the snack.

Preparation Time: 2 minutes

4. Hummus with Veggie Sticks

Ingredients:

- ➢ Hummus (store-bought or homemade)
- ➢ Assorted vegetable sticks (such as carrots, cucumber, bell peppers, celery)

Instructions:

- ➢ Spoon hummus into a small bowl or container.
- ➢ Arrange assorted vegetable sticks alongside the hummus.

➤ Dip the vegetable sticks into the hummus and enjoy as a satisfying and nutrient-rich snack.

Health Benefits:

➤ Hummus provides plant-based protein, fiber, and healthy fats, supporting hormone balance and reproductive health.

➤ Assorted vegetable sticks offer vitamins, minerals, and antioxidants, promoting overall health and fertility.

➤ This snack is convenient, portable, and perfect for on-the-go enjoyment.

Preparation Time: 5 minutes

5. Hard-Boiled Eggs with Whole Grain Crackers

Ingredients:

➤ Hard-boiled eggs
➤ Whole grain crackers

Instructions:

> Peel hard-boiled eggs and slice into halves or quarters.
> Serve alongside whole grain crackers for a nutritious and satisfying snack option.

Health Benefits:

> Hard-boiled eggs provide high-quality protein, vitamins, and minerals, supporting hormone balance and reproductive health.
> Whole grain crackers offer complex carbohydrates and fiber, sustaining energy levels and supporting reproductive function.
> This snack is simple, portable, and perfect for a quick pick-me-up during the day.

Preparation Time: 5 minutes

6. Greek Yogurt Parfait with Granola

Ingredients:

> Greek yogurt
> Mixed berries (such as strawberries, blueberries, raspberries)

➢ Granola

Instructions:

➢ In a glass or bowl, layer Greek yogurt, mixed berries, and granola.

➢ Repeat the layers until the glass or bowl is filled.

➢ Serve immediately as a nutritious and satisfying snack option.

Health Benefits:

➢ Greek yogurt provides protein, calcium, and probiotics, supporting hormone balance and reproductive health.

➢ Mixed berries offer antioxidants, vitamins, and fiber, promoting fertility and overall wellness.

➢ Granola provides complex carbohydrates and fiber, sustaining energy levels and supporting reproductive function.

Preparation Time: 5 minutes

7. Almond Butter and Banana Slices on Whole Grain Toast

Ingredients:

- Whole grain bread or toast
- Almond butter
- Ripe banana, sliced

Instructions:

- Toast whole grain bread until golden brown and crispy.
- Spread almond butter onto the toasted bread.
- Top with sliced banana.
- Serve immediately as a nutritious and satisfying snack option.

Health Benefits:

- Almond butter offers healthy fats, protein, and essential nutrients, supporting hormone balance and reproductive health.
- Whole grain bread provides complex carbohydrates and fiber, sustaining energy levels and supporting reproductive function.

> Banana offers vitamins, minerals, and fiber, promoting overall health and fertility.

Preparation Time: 5 minutes

8. Cottage Cheese with Pineapple Chunks

Ingredients:

- Cottage cheese
- Fresh pineapple, diced

Instructions:

- Spoon cottage cheese into a bowl.
- Top with diced fresh pineapple.
- Enjoy immediately as a simple and refreshing snack option.

Health Benefits:

- Cottage cheese provides protein, calcium, and essential nutrients, supporting hormone balance and reproductive health.
- Pineapple offers vitamins, minerals, and antioxidants, promoting overall health and fertility.
- This snack is light, satisfying, and perfect for a quick pick-me-up between meals.

Preparation Time: 2 minutes

9. Trail Mix with Dried Fruit and Nuts

Ingredients:

- Assorted nuts (such as almonds, cashews, walnuts)
- Dried fruit (such as apricots, cranberries, raisins)
- Optional: dark chocolate chips or chunks

Instructions:

- Combine assorted nuts, dried fruit, and optional dark chocolate chips or chunks in a bowl.
- Toss to mix evenly.
- Portion out individual servings into small containers or bags for a convenient and nutritious snack option.

Health Benefits:

- Nuts provide healthy fats, protein, and essential nutrients, supporting hormone balance and reproductive health.
- Dried fruit offers vitamins, minerals, and antioxidants, promoting overall health and fertility.

➤ Dark chocolate provides antioxidants and may offer mood-boosting benefits, enhancing the enjoyment of the snack.

Preparation Time: 5 minutes

10. Edamame with Sea Salt

Ingredients:

➤ Frozen edamame pods (shelled or unshelled)
➤ Coarse sea salt

Instructions:

➤ Cook frozen edamame according to package instructions.
➤ Drain and transfer cooked edamame to a serving bowl.
➤ Sprinkle with coarse sea salt to taste.
➤ Enjoy immediately as a nutritious and satisfying snack option.

Health Benefits:

➤ Edamame provides plant-based protein, fiber, and essential nutrients, supporting hormone balance and reproductive health.

➤ Sea salt adds flavor and may help replenish electrolytes lost through sweat, especially after physical activity.

➤ This snack is quick to prepare, convenient, and perfect for fueling up during the day.

Preparation Time: 10 minutes

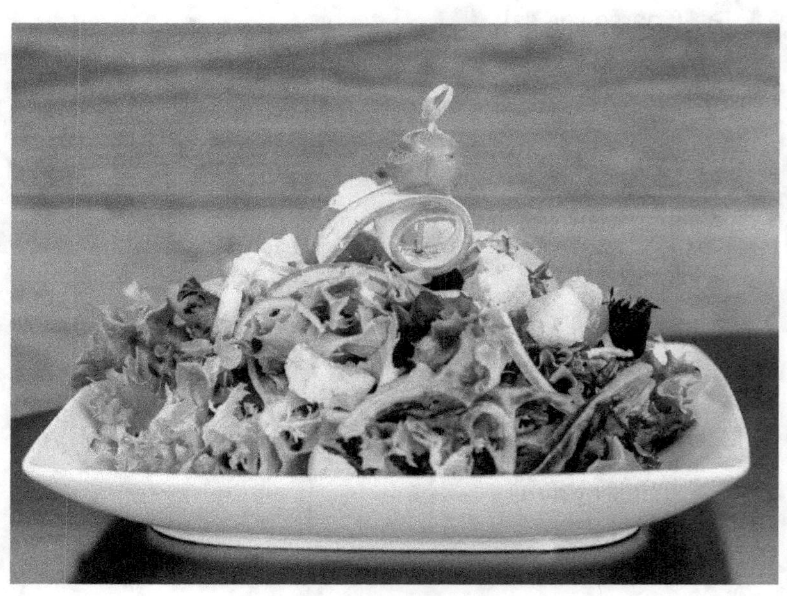

CONCLUSION

Embracing a fertility-focused diet tailored to the needs of older women can be a transformative journey towards enhancing reproductive health and increasing the chances of conception.

By prioritizing nutrient-dense foods rich in vitamins, minerals, antioxidants, and healthy fats, older women can create an optimal environment for hormonal balance, egg quality, and overall fertility.

Incorporating a variety of fruits, vegetables, whole grains, lean proteins, and plant-based fats not only nourishes the body but also supports reproductive wellness from within.

Furthermore, adopting healthy lifestyle habits such as regular exercise, stress management, and adequate hydration complements the benefits of a fertility diet, promoting overall well-being and reproductive vitality.

Consulting with healthcare providers or fertility specialists can provide personalized guidance and support, ensuring that dietary choices align with individual health needs and goals.

As older women embark on their fertility journey, it's essential to approach the process with patience, perseverance, and positivity.

While age may present unique challenges, taking proactive steps to optimize nutrition, lifestyle, and overall health can empower older women to embrace their fertility potential and pursue their dreams of conception and parenthood with confidence.

In essence, the path to fertility for older women is not just about what they eat, but also about embracing a holistic approach to wellness that nurtures the body, mind, and spirit.

With dedication, determination, and a nourishing fertility diet, older women can embark on this journey with optimism and hope, knowing that they are giving themselves the best possible chance for success.

www.ingramcontent.com/pod-product-compliance
Lightning Source LLC
Chambersburg PA
CBHW070957250726
48663CB00002B/260